TABLE OF CONTENTS

INTRODUCTION

Parkinson's disease affects nearly 1 million Americans. Each year, another 60,000 people are diagnosed with the condition. Symptoms vary from person to person but commonly include muscle spasms, tremors, and muscle soreness. The causes and triggers that activate Parkinson's are still being studied. Since Parkinson's is closely connected to a lack of dopamine cells in your body, researchers are looking for ways to increase dopamine naturally through your diet. The secondary symptoms of Parkinson's, such as dementia and confusion, might also be improved through lifestyle changes like diet and exercise. Foods high in antioxidants are sometimes suggested to cut down on oxidative stress in your brain. Levodopa (Sinemet) and bromocriptine (Parlodel) are drugs that many people with Parkinson's use to manage symptoms. But no treatment exists that will fully stop symptoms from occurring. Since there's no cure for Parkinson's, and the drugs prescribed to manage symptoms sometimes have harsh side effects, more and more people are exploring alternative remedies for Parkinson's treatment. Here's what the research says about foods to eat and avoid to help manage the symptoms of Parkinson's disease.

PARKINSON

Parkinson's disease is a progressive neurological disorder. The first signs are problems with movement. Smooth and coordinated muscle movements of the body are made possible by a substance in the brain called dopamine. Dopamine is produced in a part of the brain called the "substantia nigra." In Parkinson's, the cells of the substantia nigra start to die. When this happens, dopamine levels are reduced. When they have dropped 60 to 80 percent, symptoms of Parkinson's start to appear. There's currently no cure for Parkinson's, a disease which is chronic and worsens over time. More than 50,000 new cases are reported in the United States each year. But there may be even more, since Parkinson's is often misdiagnosed. It's reported that Parkinson's complications are the 14th major cause of death in the United States.

EARLY SIGNS OF PARKINSON'S DISEASE

Parkinson's disease (PD) is a neurological movement disorder that, according to the National Institutes of Health (NIH), affects approximately 500,000 people in the United States. Some early symptoms include:

- cramped handwriting or other writing changes

- tremor, especially in finger, hand or foot

- uncontrollable movements during sleep

- limb stiffness or slow movement (bradykinesia)

- voice changes

- rigid facial expression or masking

- stooped posture

PD starts with the brain cells, called neurons, which control movement. Neurons produce a substance called dopamine. PD sets in when the neurons die and the levels of dopamine in the brain decrease. The lack of dopamine is thought to result in the symptoms that affect the way you move. Early signs of Parkinson's disease can be easy to miss, especially if they occur sporadically. It may be time to see a doctor if you are noticing symptoms that keep appearing.

Small handwriting

A sudden change in the size of your handwriting may be an early indicator of Parkinson's disease. People with PD have a hard time controlling movement because of the changes in the brain. This can make fine motor skills like writing more difficult. Micrographia is the medical term for "small handwriting." Parkinson's patients often have handwriting that looks cramped. Individual letters tend to be smaller than normal, and words are spaced closely. A person with PD may begin writing a letter in their regular handwriting but gradually start writing in smaller font.

Tremor

Tremor is perhaps the most recognizable sign of Parkinson's disease. A slight twitching or shaking of a finger, hand, or foot is common. The person experiencing the tremor is likely to be the only person who notices them in early stages of PD. The shaking will worsen and become noticeable to others, however, as the condition progresses. The tremor is usually most noticeable at rest.

Sleep problems

Everybody has trouble sleeping from time to time. Tossing and turning takes on a new meaning when you've got Parkinson's. Early signs of the disease can include many uncontrollable movements, not just occasionally, but on a regular basis. Kicking, thrashing, flailing your arms, and even falling out of bed can be indications of a serious problem.

Stiffness and slow movement

Parkinson's disease mainly affects adults older than 60. You may feel stiff and a little slow to get going in the morning at this stage of your life. This is a completely normal development in many healthy people. The difference with PD is that the stiffness and slowness it causes don't go away as you get up and start your day. Stiffness of the limbs (rigidity) and slow movement (bradykinesia) appear early on with PD. These symptoms are caused by the impairment of the neurons that control movement. A person with PD will notice jerkier motions and move in a more uncoordinated pattern than before. Eventually, a person may develop the characteristic "shuffling gait."

Voice changes

Parkinson's disease affects movement in different ways, including how you speak. You might be familiar with the slurred speech of advanced PD patients. Less dramatic voice changes can occur in early stages of the disease. Your enunciation will most likely remain crystal clear early on in PD. You may, however, unintentionally be speaking more quietly. People in early stages of PD often speak in low tones, a hoarse voice, or with little inflection.

Masking

Parkinson's can affect the natural facial expressions in addition to gross motor skills. People often comment that some individuals with PD have a blank stare. This phenomenon, called masking, is a common sign of early PD. The disease can make movement and control of small muscles in the face difficult. Patients may have a very serious look on their face even when the conversation is lighthearted and lively. People with PD often blink less often as well.

Posture

The wide, uncontrolled, involuntary movements of Parkinson's disease don't happen overnight. Posture will change in small ways at first, and will gradually worsen. A stooped posture that can also be described as leaning and slouching is an early indicator of PD. This posture has to do with the loss of coordination and balance affecting the body. Back injuries can also cause stooping, but patients with back injuries may eventually straighten up again after a period of healing. People with PD often are unable regain that skill.

CAUSES OF PARKINSON'S DISEASE

Researchers aren't yet certain what causes Parkinson's. There are several factors that may contribute to the disease.

Genetics

Some studies suggest that genes play a role in the development of Parkinson's. An estimated 15 percent of people with Parkinson's have a family history of the condition. The Mayo Clinic reports that someone with a close relative (e.g., a parent or sibling) who has Parkinson's is at an increased risk of developing the disease. It also reports that the risk of developing Parkinson's is low unless you have several family members with the disease. How does genetics factor into Parkinson's in some families? According to Genetics Home Reference, one possible way is through the mutation of genes responsible for producing dopamine and certain proteins essential for brain function.

Environment

There's also some evidence that one's environment can play a role. Exposure to certain chemicals has been suggested as a possible link to Parkinson's disease. These include pesticides such as insecticides, herbicides, and fungicides. It's also possible that Agent Orange exposure may be linked to Parkinson's. Parkinson's has also been potentially linked to drinking well water and consuming manganese. Not everyone exposed to these environmental factors develops Parkinson's. Some researchers suspect that a combination of genetics and environmental factors cause Parkinson's.

Lewy bodies

Lewy bodies are abnormal clumps of proteins found in the brain stem of people with Parkinson's disease. These clumps contain a protein that cells are unable to break down. They surround cells in the brain. In the process they interrupt the way the brain functions. Clusters of Lewy bodies cause the brain to degenerate over time. This causes problems with motor coordination in people with Parkinson's disease.

Loss of dopamine

Dopamine is a neurotransmitter chemical that aids in passing messages between different sections of the brain. The cells that produce dopamine are damaged in people with Parkinson's disease. Without an adequate supply of dopamine the brain is unable to properly send and receive messages. This disruption affects the body's ability to co-ordinate movement. It can cause problems with walking and balance.

Age and gender

Aging also plays a role in Parkinson's disease. Advanced age is the most significant risk factor for developing

Parkinson's disease. Scientists believe that brain and dopamine function begin to decline as the body ages. This makes a person more susceptible to Parkinson's. Gender also plays a role in Parkinson's. Men are more susceptible to developing Parkinson's than women.

Occupations

Some research suggests that certain occupations may put a person at greater risk for developing Parkinson's. In particular, Parkinson's disease may be more likely for people who have jobs in welding, agriculture, and industrial work. This may be because individuals in these occupations are exposed to toxic chemicals. However, study results have been inconsistent and more research needs to be done.

PARKINSON'S DISEASE STAGES

Parkinson's disease is a progressive disease. That means symptoms of the condition typically worsen over time. Many doctors use the Hoehn and Yahr scale to classify its stages. This scale divides symptoms into five stages, and it helps healthcare providers know how advanced the disease signs and symptoms are.

Stage 1

Stage 1 Parkinson's is the mildest form. It's so mild, in fact, you may not experience symptoms that are noticeable. They may not yet interfere with your daily life and tasks. If you do have symptoms, they may be isolated to one side of your body.

Stage 2

The progression from stage 1 to stage 2 can take months, or even years. Each person's experience will be different. At this moderate stage, you may experience symptoms such as:

• muscle stiffness

• tremors

• changes in facial expressions

• trembling

Muscle stiffness can complicate daily tasks, prolonging how long it takes you to complete them. However, at this stage, you're unlikely to experience balance problems. Symptoms may appear on both sides of the body. Changes in posture, gait, and facial expressions may be more noticeable.

Stage 3

At this middle stage, symptoms reach a turning point. While you're unlikely to experience new symptoms, they may be more noticeable. They may also interfere with all of your daily tasks. Movements are noticeably slower, which slows down activities. Balance issues become more significant, too, so falls are more common. But people with stage 3 Parkinson's can usually maintain their independence and complete activities without much assistance.

Stage 4

The progression from stage 3 to stage 4 brings about significant changes. At this point, you will experience great difficulty standing without a walker or assistive device. Reactions and muscle movements also slow significantly. Living alone can be unsafe, possibly dangerous.

Stage 5

In this most advanced stage, severe symptoms make around-the-clock assistance a necessity. It will be difficult to stand, if not impossible. A wheelchair will likely be required. Also, at this stage, individuals with Parkinson's may experience confusion, delusions, and hallucinations.

These complications of the disease can begin in the later stages. This is the most common Parkinson's disease stage system, but alternative staging systems for Parkinson's are sometimes used.

DIAGNOSING PARKINSON'S DISEASE

There's no specific test for diagnosing Parkinson's. Diagnosis is made based on health history, a physical and neurological exam, as well as a review of signs and symptoms. Imaging tests, such as a CAT scan or MRI, may be used to rule out other conditions. A dopamine transporter (DAT) scan may also be used. While these tests don't confirm Parkinson's, they can help rule out other conditions and support the doctor's diagnosis.

TREATMENTS FOR PARKINSON'S DISEASE

Treatment for Parkinson's relies on a combination of lifestyle changes, medications, and therapies. Adequate rest, exercise, and a balanced diet are important. Speech therapy, occupational therapy, and physical therapy can also help to improve communication and self-care. In almost all cases, medication will be required to help control the various physical and mental health symptoms associated with the disease.

DRUGS AND MEDICATION USED TO TREAT PARKINSON'S DISEASE

A number of different drugs can be used to treat Parkinson's.

Levodopa: Levodopa is the most common treatment for Parkinson's. It helps to replenish dopamine. About 75 percent of cases respond to levodopa, but not all symptoms are improved. Levodopa is generally given with carbidopa. Carbidopa delays the breakdown of levodopa which in turn increases the availability of levodopa at the blood-brain barrier.

Dopamine agonists: Dopamine agonists can imitate the action of dopamine in the brain. They're less effective than levodopa, but they can be useful as bridge medications when levodopa is less effective. Drugs in this class include bromocriptine, pramipexole, and ropinirole.

Anticholinergics: Anticholinergics are used to block the

parasympathetic nervous system. They can help with rigidity. Benztropine (Cogentin) and trihexyphenidyl are anticholinergics used to treat Parkinson's.

Amantadine (Symmetrel): Amantadine (Symmetrel) can be used along with carbidopa-levodopa. It's a glutamate blocking drug (NMDA). It offers short-term relief for the involuntary movements (dyskinesia) that can be a side effect of levodopa.

COMT inhibitors: Catechol O-methyltransferase (COMT) inhibitors prolong the effect of levodopa. Entacapone (Comtan) and tolcapone (Tasmar) are examples of COMT inhibitors. Tolcapone can cause liver damage. It's usually saved for people who don't respond to other therapies. Ectacapone doesn't cause liver damage. Stalevo is a drug that combines ectacapone and carbidopa-levodopa in one pill.

MAO B inhibitors: MAO B inhibitors inhibit the enzyme monoamine oxidase B. This enzyme breaks down dopamine in the brain. Selegiline (Eldepryl) and rasagiline (Azilect) are examples of MAO B inhibitors. Talk with your doctor before taking any other medications with MAO B inhibitors. They can interact with many drugs, including:

- antidepressants

- ciprofloxacin

- St. John's wort

- some narcotics

Over time, the effectiveness of Parkinson's medications can decrease. By late-stage Parkinson's, the side effects of some medicines may outweigh the benefits. However, they may still provide adequate control of symptoms.

Parkinson's Surgery

Surgical interventions are reserved for people who don't respond to medication, therapy, and lifestyle changes. Two primary types of surgery are used to treat Parkinson's:

Deep brain stimulation

During deep brain stimulation (DBS), surgeons implant electrodes in specific parts of the brain. A generator connected to the electrodes sends out pulses to help reduce symptoms.

Pump-delivered therapy

In January 2015, the U.S. Food and Drug Administration (FDA) approved a pump-delivered therapy called Duopa. The pump delivers a combination of levodopa and carbidopa. In order to use the pump, your doctor will have to perform a surgical procedure to place the pump near the small intestine.

PARKINSON'S PROGNOSIS

Complications from Parkinson's can greatly reduce quality of life and prognosis. For example, individuals with Parkinson's can experience dangerous falls, as well as blood clots in the lungs and legs. These complications can be fatal. Proper treatment improves your prognosis, and it increases life expectancy. It may not be possible to slow the progression of Parkinson's, but you can work to overcome the obstacles and complications to have a better quality of life for as long as possible.

PARKINSON'S PREVENTION

Doctors and researchers don't understand what causes Parkinson's. They're also not sure why it progresses differently in each person. That's why it's unclear how you can prevent the disease. Each year, researchers investigate why Parkinson's occurs and what can be done to prevent it. Recent research suggests lifestyle factors — like physical exercise and a diet rich in antioxidants — may have a protective effect. If you have a family history of Parkinson's, you may consider genetic testing. Certain genes have been connected to Parkinson's. But it's important to know that having these gene mutations does not mean you'll definitely develop the disease. Talk to your doctor about the risks and benefits of genetic testing.

PARKINSON'S HEREDITY

Researchers believe both your genes and the environment may play a role in whether or not you get Parkinson's. How great their impact can be, however, is unknown. Most cases occur in people with no apparent family history of the disease. Hereditary cases of Parkinson's are rare. It's uncommon for parents to pass Parkinson's to a child. According to the National Institutes of Health, only 15 percent of people with Parkinson's have a family history of the disease.

PARKINSON'S DEMENTIA

Parkinson's dementia is a complication of Parkinson's disease. It causes people to develop difficulties with reasoning, thinking, and problem solving. It's quite common — 50 to 80 percent of people with Parkinson's will experience some degree of dementia. Symptoms of Parkinson's disease dementia include:

- depression

- sleep disturbances

- delusions

- confusion

- hallucinations

- mood swings

- slurred speech

- changes in appetite

- changes in energy level

Parkinson's disease destroys chemical-receiving cells in the brain. Over time, this can lead to dramatic changes, symptoms, and complications. Certain people are more likely to develop Parkinson's disease dementia. Risk factors for the condition include:

• Sex: Men are more likely to develop it.

• Age: The risk increases as you get older.

• Existing cognitive impairment: If you had memory and mood issues before a Parkinson's diagnosis, your risk may be higher for dementia.

• Severe Parkinson's symptoms: You may be more at risk for Parkinson's disease dementia if you have severe motor impairment, such as rigid muscles and difficulty walking.

Currently, there's no treatment for Parkinson's disease dementia. Instead, a doctor will focus on treating other symptoms. Sometimes medications used for other types of dementia can be helpful.

PARKINSON'S LIFE EXPECTANCY

Parkinson's disease is not fatal. However, Parkinson's-related complications can shorten the lifespan of people diagnosed with the disease. Having Parkinson's increases a person's risk for potentially life-threatening complications, like a fall, blood clots, lung infections, and blockages in the lungs. These complications can cause severe health issues. They can even be fatal. It's unclear how much Parkinson's reduces a person's life expectancy. One study looked at the 6-year survival rates of nearly 140,000 people who had been diagnosed with Parkinson's. In that six-year span 64 percent of people with Parkinson's died. What's more, the study found that 70 percent of people in the study had been diagnosed with Parkinson's disease dementia during the span of the study. Those who were diagnosed with the memory disorder had lower survival rates.

Parkinson's Exercises

Parkinson's often causes problems with daily activities. But very simple exercises and stretches may help you move around and walk more safely.

To improve walking

• Walk carefully.

- Pace yourself—try not to move too quickly.

- Let your heel hit the floor first.

- Check your posture and stand up straight. This will help you to shuffle less.

To avoid falling

- Don't walk backwards.

- Try to not carry things while walking.

- Try to avoid leaning and reaching.

- To turn around, make a U-turn. Don't pivot on your feet.

- Remove all tripping hazards in your house such as loose rugs.

When getting dressed

- Allow yourself plenty of time to get ready. Avoid rushing.

- Select clothes that are easy to put on and take off.

- Try using items with Velcro instead of buttons.

- Try wearing pants and skirts with elastic waist bands. These may be easier than buttons and zippers.

Yoga uses targeted muscle movement to build muscle, increase mobility, and improve flexibility. People with Parkinson's may notice yoga even helps control tremors in some affected limbs.

PARKINSON'S AND DOPAMINE

Parkinson's disease is a neurodegenerative disorder. It affects the dopamine-producing neurons (dopaminergic) in the brain. Dopamine is a brain chemical and neurotransmitter. It helps send electric signals around the brain and through the body. The disease prevents these cells from making dopamine, and it may impair how well the brain can use dopamine. Over time, the cells will die entirely. The drop in dopamine is often gradual. That's why symptoms progress, or slowly get worse. Many of the Parkinson's medications are dopaminergic drugs. They aim to increase the level of dopamine or make it more effective on the brain.

PARKINSON'S VS MS

At first glance, Parkinson's disease and multiple sclerosis (MS) may seem very similar. They both affect the central nervous system, and they can produce many similar symptoms. These include:

- tremors

- slurred speech

- poor balance and instability

- changes in movement and gait

- muscle weakness or loss of muscle coordination

The two conditions are very different, however. The key differences include:

Cause

MS is an autoimmune disorder. Parkinson's is the result of decreased dopamine levels in the brain.

Age

MS primarily affects younger individuals. Average age of diagnosis is between 20 and 50. Parkinson's is more common in people over 60.

Symptoms

People with MS experience issues like headaches, hearing loss, pain, and double vision. Parkinson's can ultimately cause muscle rigidity and difficulty walking, poor posture, loss of muscle control, hallucinations, and dementia. If you're showing unusual symptoms, your doctor may consider both of these conditions when making a diagnosis. Imaging tests and blood tests may be able to help distinguish between the two conditions.

PARKINSON DIET

Foods To Eat

Antioxidants

Current research focuses on proteins, flavonoids, and gut bacteria for improving Parkinson's symptoms. In the meantime, eating a diet high in antioxidants reduces "oxidative stress" that aggravates Parkinson's and similar conditions, according to the Michael J. Fox Foundation for Parkinson's research. You can get lots of antioxidants by eating:

• tree nuts, like walnuts, Brazil nuts, pecans, and pistachios

• blueberries, blackberries, goji berries, cranberries, and elderberries

• tomatoes, peppers, eggplant, and other nightshade vegetables

• spinach and kale

Eating a plant-based diet high in these types of foods may provide the highest antioxidant intake. Clinical trials over the last decade explored the idea of antioxidant treatment for Parkinson's, but these trials didn't find concrete evidence to link antioxidants to Parkinson's treatment. But decreasing oxidative stress is still a simple way to improve your lifestyle and get healthier. In other words, it can't hurt.

Fava beans

Some people eat fava beans for Parkinson's because they contain levodopa — the same ingredient in some drugs used to treat Parkinson's. There's no definitive evidence supporting fava beans as a treatment at this time. Since you don't know how much levodopa you're getting when you eat fava beans, they can't substitute for prescription treatments.

Omega-3s

If you're concerned about secondary symptoms of Parkinson's, like dementia and confusion, get serious about consuming more salmon, halibut, oysters, soybeans, flax seed, and kidney beans. Soy in particular is being studied for its ability to protect against Parkinson's. These foods contain omega-3 fatty acids, which might improve cognitive function.

OTHER TIPS

• For constipation caused by Parkinson's, try seasoning your food with turmeric or yellow mustard to encourage bowel movements.

• One study suggested that consuming caffeine might help slow down the progression of Parkinson's.

• For muscle cramps caused by Parkinson's, consider drinking tonic water for the quinine it contains or upping your magnesium through diet, Epsom salt baths, or supplements.

FOODS TO AVOID

Dairy products

Dairy products have been linked to a risk of developing Parkinson's. Something in dairy products might negatively impact the oxidation levels in your brain, making symptoms more persistent. This effect was shown to be stronger in men than in women and not seen in those supplementing with calcium. If you're going to stop consuming dairy products like milk, cheese, and yogurt, you might want to consider a calcium supplement to make up for the loss of calcium in your diet. However, low calcium intake doesn't necessarily equal poor bone health, as seen in countries with low dairy and calcium consumption. Recent research suggests that a defect in how the body manages calcium ions (Ca2+), the form of calcium residing in bone, and also present in dairy, might be to blame for the progression of Parkinson's disease.

Foods high in saturated fat

The role that foods high in saturated fats play in Parkinson's progression is still under investigation and is often conflicting. We might eventually discover that there are certain types of saturated fats that actually help people with Parkinson's. Some limited research does show that ketogenic, low-protein diets were beneficial for some with Parkinson's. Other research finds high saturated fat intake worsened risk. But in general, foods that have been fried or heavily processed alter your metabolism, increase blood pressure, and impact your cholesterol. None of those things are good for your body, especially if you're trying to treat Parkinson's.

LIFESTYLE TIPS

Staying hydrated is important for everyone, especially people with Parkinson's. Aim to drink six to eight glasses of water each day to feel your best. Vitamin D has been demonstrated to protect against Parkinson's, so getting fresh air and sunshine might help your symptoms, too. Different kinds of exercise and physical therapy can improve your abilities and slow the progression of Parkinson's. Talk to you doctor about supplements you might take and exercises that would be safe for you to try.

ONE-DAY MEAL PLAN

When chewing takes a long time, small, frequent meals and snacks may be better than three large meals a day. It also helps to take small bites. As a soft-food diet is more limited, it may be advisable to use fortified foods and a multivitamin-mineral supplement. Although chewing problems require adjustments in cooking and serving foods, it is important to have a varied, healthy, and nourishing daily meal plan. This will help to get the vital nutrients needed, and enough calories to maintain a healthy weight. Here is an example of a carefully chosen one-day menu with all the flavour, vitamins, minerals, and fibre you need, featuring the salmon recipe above.

NOTE: If the portions are too small, increase as needed.

Breakfast:

- 177ml calcium-fortified orange juice

- 220g cooked oatmeal

- 30g raisins

- 120ml 1% fat milk or calcium-fortified milk alternative

- Coffee or tea

Snack:

- 12ml apple sauce

- 1 scrambled egg

Tip: You may crush a multivitamin tablet and mix into the apple sauce.

Lunch:

- 235ml split pea soup

- 1 whole-grain rye crisp biscuit/cracker, crumbled and added to the soup to soften

- 30g cheese or vegan cheese, grated and added to the soup

- 220g bread pudding or rice pudding (made with milk alternative if needed, and whole- grain bread or brown rice)

- 175ml tomato juice

Dinner:

- Salmon and vegetable potato topper

- 110g mashed turnips or cooked finely chopped spinach

- 240g milk or milk alternative, or coffee or tea as preferred

- 1 poached pear, chopped

Recipes

Vegetarian 'Beet Wellington' With Mushrooms, Aubergines And Garlic

Rich in fibre and low in protein, this 'Beet Wellington' – a vegetarian spin-off of a steak classic – is a delicious combination of beetroots, mushrooms, aubergines and garlic.

Ingredients

- 140g fresh, organic beetroots

- 100g mushrooms

- 4 sheets 20x20cm puff pastry

- 3 tbsp breadcrumbs

- 2 shallots (roughly chopped)

- 2 pinches of aniseed

- 1 clove of garlic (roughly chopped)

- 1 tbsp of cut sage

- 1 tbsp tomato purée

- 1 aubergine (diced)

- 1 egg yolk (mixed with 1 tbsp oil and water)

- 1 tsp poppy seeds (optional)

- Sunflower oil

- Flour

- Pepper

- Salt (optional)

Method

- Preheat oven to 180°C.

- Place the beetroots into an oven dish and brush them with sunflower oil.

- Roast the beetroots in the oven for 45 minutes.

- Remove the skin from the beetroots.

- Mix sunflower oil with pepper, 1 pinch of aniseed and

sage.

• Brush the oil mixture onto the beetroots. Sprinkle some salt on top (optional).

• Heat sunflower oil in a frying pan and fry the aubergine, shallots, garlic and mushrooms.

• Add the tomato purée and a splash of water, stir thoroughly.

• Add the breadcrumbs, sage and 1 pinch of aniseed. Cook on a low heat for ten minutes, stirring from time to time.

• Purée the mixture in a blender, leave to cool.

• Pre-heat the oven to 220°C.

• Place sheets of pastry on a cool, floured surface.

• Brush the edges of the pastry with the mixture of egg yolk, water and oil.

• Place ½ tbsp of breadcrumbs in the middle of each sheet.

• Spread the purée mixture over the sheets of pastry.

• Place the beetroot on top of the purée mixture.

• As tightly as possible, fold the pastry sheets over the purée and beetroot.

• Turn the pastry over and brush egg yolk over the top.

• Sprinkle poppy seeds over the dough (optional).

• Bake the Beet Wellington for 20 minutes, until golden brown.

Culinary tip: Serve with a cool, homemade sauce comprising of sour cream, horseradish and a splash of vodka.

Variation: You can replace the beetroot with a large turnip of half a kohlrabi.

Colourful Broccoli, Shiitake Mushrooms And Cashew Nut Stir-Fry

Make your own vegetarian stir-fry with broccoli, shiitakes and cashew nuts. This recipe is packed with fibre, protein and is also easy to digest

Ingredients

• 2 eggs

• 300g broccoli florets

• 240g thin Chinese egg noodles (boiled)

• 200g baby corn cobs

• 100g shiitake mushrooms

• 100g cashew nuts (coarsely chopped)

• 4 tbsp oil

• 2 tbsp water

• 2 tbsp ginger syrup

• 2 tbsp lemon juice

• 2 tbsp sunflower oil

• 1 tbsp sesame oil

• 2 cloves of garlic (thinly sliced)

• 1 red onion, sliced into rings

Method

• Remove the stalks from the shiitakes and cut the tops

into quarters.

• Blanch the baby corn for two minutes and then the broccoli for one minute.

• Fry both the onion and garlic in a wok.

• Add the shiitake mushrooms and fry for one minute on a high heat.

• Add the baby corn and broccoli.

• Add the water, ginger syrup and lemon juice. Heat for a further two minutes.

• Add the nuts.

• Fry the egg noodles in a mixture of sunflower and sesame oil.

• Beat the eggs and stir into the noodles.

Culinary tip: Instead of water, use a splash of Thai chilli or soy sauce for different flavours.

Variation tip: For a non-vegetarian option, use Norwegian prawns or pre-cooked strips of chicken.

Rich Chocolate Fondue With Strawberries And Pineapple

Make your own chocolate fondue with a selection of delicious fruits. This meal is full of fibre and easy to digest, suitable for those with chewing difficulties

Ingredients

• 300g pure chocolate (70% cocoa)

• 250g washed strawberries

• 250g fresh pineapple, diced and dried

- 100ml whipped cream

- 4 slices of cake

Method

- Warm the chocolate with the cream in a bowl, using the bain-marie method, while stirring into a smooth sauce.

- Place a fondue hot plate on the table and light the candle below. Put the pan with chocolate sauce on top of the plate.

- Skewer a piece of fruit on a fork and dip into the chocolate sauce.

Bread Rosettes With Spinach, Feta And Oregano

Make your own bread substitute with the addition of delicious and healthy vegetables. This dish is rich in fiber and it's also soft, making it easy to digest

Ingredients

For 12 rosettes

- 500g whole wheat flour

- 500g spinach leaves

- 200g crumbled feta

- 20g fresh or 2 packets of dry yeast

- 2 tsp dried oregano

- 2 tbsp olive oil

- 250ml water (lukewarm)

- 2 cloves of garlic (coarsely chopped)

- 4 tbsp olive oil

• pinch of salt

Method

• Put the flour in a mixing bowl. Add the fresh, crumbled yeast or dried yeast and mix through the flour.

• Mix in 1 tsp of oregano. Make a well in the center and pour in the olive oil and water. Mix until a soft dough form. Add the salt. Leave to rest for 15 minutes.

• Knead the dough for 5–10 minutes until supple and elastic.

• Form a ball, place it in the mixing bowl, cover with cling film and allow to rise in a warm spot for 1 hour, or until the volume has doubled.

• Fry the garlic in olive oil at low heat until glazed. Turn the heat up and add the spinach. Allow to cook and turn over from time to time.

• Use a strainer to remove all the water from the spinach.

• Apply olive oil to the work surface.

• Roll the dough into a 50 x 30cm rectangle with a thickness of 0.75cm.

• Divide the spinach and feta over the dough.

• Make a loose roll, starting at a short side.

• Cut the roll of dough into 12 slices and place the slices on a baking tray covered with baking paper.

• Cover with a floured towel and allow to rise for 1 hour.

• Pre-heat the oven at 200°C and bake the bread in 20–25 minutes until golden brown.

- Allow the bread to cool on a grid outside the oven.

Culinary tip: Why not make a tasty sauce by seasoning crème fraiche with chopped basil and thick balsamic vinegar.

Variation: This dish also works well if you replace the spinach with braised chard. Divide the chard into leaves and stalks, then cut into small pieces and blanch.

Sicilian Caponata: Aubergines In A 'Puttanesca' Tomato Sauce

A delicious lunch dish packed full of fibre and robust flavours. It's ideal for people who are sensitive to protein and it's soft making it easily digestible

Ingredients

- 2 aubergines (diced)

- 2 onions (coarsely chopped)

- 3 celery stalks (peeled and diced)

- 3 tbsp olive oil

- 2 plum tomatoes (finely chopped)

- 2 cloves of garlic (thin slices)

- 3 celery stalks (peeled and diced)

- 2 beefsteak tomatoes (diced)

- 1 red bell pepper (finely chopped)

- 12 black, pitted olives (coarsely chopped)

- 2 tbsp green herbs

- 2 tbsp jam sugar

- 1 tbsp white wine vinegar

- ½ tbsp small capers

- 1 tsp paprika

- cayenne pepper

- salt and pepper

Method

Sicilian Caponata

- Place the diced aubergine into salted cold water for 10 minutes.

- Gently dry the diced aubergine.

- Fry the aubergine with the onion in olive oil.

- Add the garlic and the celery and braise for 3 minutes.

- Add the tomatoes, olives, capers and the sugar.

- Deglaze with white wine vinegar.

- Season with salt, pepper and cayenne pepper.

- Leave to cool and mix in the green herbs.

Putanesca sauce

- Fry the onion and bell pepper in olive oil.

- Add the tomatoes.

- Season with salt, pepper and paprika.

- Allow the ingredients to cook thoroughly.

- Add water if the sauce becomes too thick.

- Pass the sauce through a sieve and leave to cool

Culinary tip: The sauce tastes best when it's nice and spicy. Garnish the caponata with pickled anchovies. This salad is also very suitable side for a barbecue.

Leftovers tip: Warm up the salad the following day for lunch or use as a side for a dish with lamb or chicken.

Variation: This dish is effectively an alternative ratatouille; you can experiment with adding or leaving out ingredients of your choice.

Indonesian Minced Pork With Caramelized Pumpkin And Cucumber Soup

This Asian-inspired dish combines soft minced pork and honey-caramelized pumpkin, served with a cooling cucumber soup. The recipe can be adapted for people with chewing or swallowing problems – without losing the intense flavors.

Ingredients

Stewed pumpkin with egg

- 240g brown wholegrain rice

- 400g pumpkin

- 400g pork mince

- 4 eggs

- 2 tbsp soy sauce

- 1 tbsp honey or agave syrup

- 100ml olive oil

- 4 cloves garlic

- fresh ginger (a small piece)

Cucumber soup

- 2 cucumbers (large)

- 1l chicken or vegetable stock

- 2 onions

- salt and pepper

- fresh coriander or parsley

Preparation

- Peel the cucumbers and cut into chunks. Remove the seeds from the pumpkin and dice.

- Peel the onion and cut into slices.

- Peel the ginger and cut into medium-sized chunks.

- Mix the garlic and the ginger into the olive oil – this mixture will form the base of the stew.

- Boil the rice and leave to drain.

Method – cucumber soup

- Fry the onion in a medium-sized saucepan in two tablespoons of the olive oil mixture.

- Add the chicken stock and bring to the boil.

- Add the cucumber and mix well.

- Season with salt and pepper.

Method – stewed pumpkin with egg

- Soft boil the eggs.

- Fry the pumpkin cubes and the pork mince in a pan in two tablespoons of the olive oil mixture.

- Add the honey and gently caramelize.

- Add the soy sauce and stew until cooked.

Variation and serving tip

- Option 1: use chicken or minced beef and fry with the pumpkin. You could also leave out the meat and use an extra egg.

- Option 2: serve the rice with the pumpkin mix and a boiled egg together in a cup of hot cucumber soup, garnish the soup with parsley or coriander.

- Option 2: serve the soup and the pumpkin separately; you can mix the coriander or parsley with a dash of oil as a garnish.

Salmon And Vegetable Potato Topper

Ingredients

- 350ml milk or milk alternative

- 230g thinly sliced carrots, cooked and drained

- 230g canned salmon, drained

- 90g grated Cheddar cheese or vegan cheese

- 4 tbsp minced onion

- 4 tbsp minced bell peppers

- 2 tbsp unsalted butter

- 1 1/2 tbsp whole wheat flour

- 1/4 teaspoon garlic powder

- 1/8 teaspoon ground thyme

- ground marjoram

• pre-baked potatoes

Method

• In a medium-sized saucepan, sauté the onion and bell peppers in butter for five minutes or until vegetables are tender.

• Combine the flour, garlic powder, thyme and marjoram. Stir into onion mixture. Heat and stir for one or two minutes.

• Remove from heat. Slowly stir in the milk or milk alternative.

• Return to heat and stir until the sauce becomes thickened and reaches the boil.

• Stir in the cheese, cooked carrots and salmon and heat through.

• Split the baked potatoes and fluff the insides with a fork. Discard the potato skins.

• Spoon the salmon mixture over potatoes and stir lightly to blend with and moisten the potato.

Greek-Inspired Courgette And Aubergine Vegetarian Moussaka

The chefs at Parki's Kookatelier have taken a Greek classic and transformed it into a vegetarian delight. What's more, it can be adapted for people with chewing and/or swallowing problems

Ingredients

• 1kg firm potatoes

• 30g soy butter

- 40g wheat flour

- 700ml unsweetened soy milk

- 500g tofu (or seitan)

- 8 fresh tomatoes (or 1 tin of tomatoes)

- 3 garlic cloves

- 1 aubergine

- 1 courgette

- 1 sweet pepper

- 1 onion

- 1 tsp oregano

- nutmeg

- salt and pepper

- olive oil

Preparation

- Preheat the oven to 180°C.

- Boil the potatoes until 'al dente' and cut into slices.

- Slice the aubergine, courgette and sweet pepper. Dice the tomato.

Method

- For the white sauce: melt the soy butter and mix with the flour. Stir well with a wooden ladle until the roux is dry.

- Pour the soy milk into the sauce little by little, while stirring with a whisk until it becomes a smooth, firm sauce. NB – you could also bind the soy milk with a white sauce binding agent.

• Season with salt, pepper and nutmeg and boil for a few more minutes while stirring.

• For the tomato sauce, fry the onions in heated olive oil until glazed.

• Add the tofu or seitan and stew for another five minutes on a low heat.

• Add oregano, garlic and tomato, bring to the boil while stirring, leave to simmer for 10 minutes.

• Place the aubergine, courgettes and the sweet pepper onto a greased oven dish and put into the oven. NB – you could also fry the vegetables on both sides in a pan with olive oil.

Taste tip: Tofu is a meat replacement made of soy milk. It has a bland flavor but easily takes up the flavors of other foods. It is low in fat and rich in proteins. When cut it into cubes, tofu is easy to shallow fry, deep fry and grill. Seitan is a wheat gluten meal replacement.

Finishing

• Put a layer of vegetables into a lightly greased deep oven dish. Next, add a layer of potatoes and a layer of tomato sauce.

• Finish with the white sauce.

• Put the moussaka into the oven for another 15 minutes.

Broccoli And Salmon Crustless Quiche

This delicious dish can be made using whatever vegetables happen to be in season and, as it's high in protein, it's a great healthy option. It can also be modified for people with chewing and/or swallowing problems

Ingredients

- 400g broccoli florets (fresh or frozen)
- 400g smoked salmon
- 3ml cream or soy cream
- 50g grated Emmental cheese
- 3 eggs
- 1 extra yolk
- 1 tbsp dill
- salt and pepper
- cayenne pepper
- nutmeg

Preparation

- 1.Break the broccoli into florets, cut the salmon into fine strips, and chop the dill.
- 2. Preheat the oven to 180 °C.

Method

- Cook the broccoli in lightly salted water, pour into a sieve and rinse immediately in cold running water to preserve its dark green color. Drain well.
- Mix the cream, eggs and herbs, spices and seasoning.
- Finely chop the broccoli florets.
- Grease or line a baking mould.
- Spread the broccoli on the bottom of the tin with a layer

of salmon strips on the top.

- Fill the moulds three-quarters with the cream mixture.

- Sprinkle with grated cheese.

- Bake for 25 minutes at 180°C.

- Leave the quiche on a cooling rack. Once cool, take the moulds away and put on a plate.

Taste tip

- For alternative flavours, use ham or leek instead of salmon.

- The quiche can be eaten both warm and cold.

Chicory With Ham And Cheese Sauce

When cooked, chicory's sharp flavour softens into a mellow sweetness and cuts through the rich ham – delicious. This recipe can be adapted especially for people with chewing and/or swallowing problems

Ingredients

- 600g potatoes

- 200g gruyere cheese (grated)

- 50g parmesan cheese (grated)

- 700ml semi-skimmed milk

- 8 chicory heads (ground)

- 8 slices cooked ham

- 50g butter

- 40g flour

- 1/2 lemon

- 1 tsp white sugar

- salt and pepper

- nutmeg

Preparation

- Clean the chicory, remove the outer leaves and the hard core.

- Cut the chicory into fine rings.

- Peel and cut the potatoes for the purée.

- Roll up the slices of ham and cut them finely.

Method

- Stew the chicory in 20g of butter with sugar, salt, pepper and nutmeg until cooked. Leave to drain and reserve the cooking liquid.

- Boil the potatoes, mash and season with salt, pepper and nutmeg.

- Prepare a béchamel sauce with a roux made from 30g butter and 40g flour. Deglaze the roux with the cold milk and stir firmly with a whisk to prevent clotting.

Tip: You can also prepare the sauce with a white sauce binder. Season with the preserved cooking liquid of the chicory, pepper, salt and nutmeg.

Finishing

- Add ¾ of the cheese to the béchamel sauce and the juice of half a lemon.

- Lightly butter a casserole dish.

• First put the puree in, then the chicory, on top the ham and finally the cheese sauce.

• Sprinkle the remainder of the grated cheese over the top and gratinate under the grill.

• Garnish with slices of lemon.

Rich Roast Pork Orloff With Vegetables And Red Pesto

French 'master chef' Urbain Dubois – who was in the employ of Prince Orloff, former Russian ambassador to France – 'discovered' the red meat dish in the mid-19th century. Over time it has been adapted to personal tastes and this particular recipe has been adapted especially for people with chewing and/or swallowing problems

Ingredients

• 600g pork (boneless ribs)

• 6 slices of cooked ham

• 200g grated cheese (Emmental or Gruèyre)

• 500ml brown cream sauce

• 200g mushrooms

• 1 glass white wine

• 2 tbsp olive oil

• 1 tbsp red pesto

• 1 tsp paprika powder

• 1 tbsp lemon juice

• 2 cloves garlic

• 2 carrots

- 1 onion

- 1 knob of butter

Preparation

- Preheat the oven to 180°C.

- Chop the carrots, onion, and the garlic into small pieces and slice the mushrooms.

- Cut the pork lengthwise – but don't cut completely through.

- Season the inside of the pork with salt, pepper, paprika and rub with red pesto.

- Place the slices of ham on top of the pork and layer with grated cheese.

- Roll the roast tightly, press firmly and tie with twine.

Method

- Place the meat in a greased roasting tin and roast in the preheated oven for 40 minutes – regularly basting with the juices.

- Meanwhile, fry the chopped onions, carrots and garlic in a pan, without browning. Add the mushrooms and sprinkle with lemon juice.

- Stew the vegetables until al-dente.

- Deglaze with the white wine and reduce until most of the liquid has evaporated.

Finishing

- Take the dish out of the oven, remove the roasting fat and carve into thick slices.

• Place the slices back into the roasting tin and pour the brown cream sauce over the stewed vegetables.

• Put the complete dish back into the oven and roast at 120 °C for a final five minutes.